WILDERNESS SURVIVAL

Stay Safe In the Wild and Learn How to Survive Anywhere (The Ultimate Guide to Survival Strategies and Tricks)

By JULIAN DRESDEN

Table of Contents

Introduction

Are you planning a trip to a destination you've never been and you want to be sure you know how to survive if there is an emergency?

Are you looking for a survival book that tells you how to survive without using manmade goods and just the clothes on your back and the natural items around you?

Then you've found that book!

Wilderness Survival: Stay Safe in the Wild and Learn How to Survive Anywhere (The Ultimate Guide to Survival Strategies and Tricks) will teach you how to survive in the wilderness anywhere and how to signal for help if you are in a tough situation. You'll learn how to find food, water, shelter, create a fire without matches, and how to signal for help so that you can survive in the wilderness.

In this book, you will learn:

- The five different ways to find water in the wilderness.
- Two ways to filter the water and make it safe for drinking by using the materials around you.
- The best thing you can eat in the wilderness and how to test new and strange foliage to see if it's edible.

- How to light a fire several different ways without the use of matches, water bottles, or any other manmade product.
- Several different types of shelters you can build depend on your situation.
- And how to signal for help in a few different ways in order to bring yourself back to civilization.

Survival is a key component of human instinct, but without the basic knowledge of how to find the five key elements to survival, you lack a great advantage.

Chapter One – Finding and Securing a Source of Water

For the sake of argument, let's say you're in the wild without a water bottle. Let's say you have nothing on you that could hold water, and so you have to find fresh water on a daily basis in order to survive. Finding water is not as difficult as it might seem. In fact, if you find yourself in the dessert, simply remove your shoes and start stepping around. It's a fact that the human feet are very sensitive to temperature differences and the feel of water, so they're a great divining rod! Just make sure you don't keep your shoes off too long or your feet will start to sweat and you'll lose more water from your body.

If you don't want to walk around barefoot and you're in a wooded area, then you simply have to look a little and use some common sense. Think about it, there has to be water around somewhere if the trees are flourishing.

If you can't seem to find a water source, begin walking downhill and keep an eye out for dark patches in the landscape. Also, look for vegetation that stands out in a low area. If you're traveling through a dessert, you might want to plan ahead of time to be sure you know where water sources are. If you do a little planning, you won't find yourself in your own personal reality show where you have to do untoward things.

Once you find a water source, determine what type it is.

Clear, Flowing Water: If your water source is coming from the somewhere void of people, manmade structures, or obvious signs of pollution, then it's most likely safe to drink without having to purify it. If you come across a stream or a spring while you're outdoors and you happen to have a water bottle, top it off. If you don't have one, rest assured there will most likely be another one on your journey through the woods.

Ponds, Lakes, and Rivers: These are less than ideal sources of water. Ponds and lakes are stagnant sources of water, which can increase the levels of bacteria, viruses, and pollution. In addition, large rivers might seem like a good source and look fresh, but they're usually full of pollution. Be very wary if there has been any recent flooding in the area if the river flows through a populated area, under a road, or around construction or other types of manmade structures.

Ice and Snow: Snow and ice, as long as it's not the ice from the ocean, will provide you with a readily available, good source of clean water in the winter time. Do not eat the snow or ice because it will lower your body temperature and you have to eat a lot of it to stay hydrated. It's much better to find a way to melt it down if you can. You still should purify snow before you drink it and be sure it's not yellow, black, or brown. To melt the snow, you can put it in a container with a little water in the bottom and bring it up to the water's temperature, adding more snow as it melts. If you don't have a container and you have no way of bringing it to a liquid state, eat it slowly in order to avoid shocking your body.

Dry River Bed or Low Lying Area: Some other options include digging a well about ten feet away from a river or a low lying area and seeing if water bubbles up. If it does, you can drink the mud water or you can run it through your shirt with some sand to make it taste a little better.

Foliage: Lastly, you can always take a look around for foliage that has moisture in it. All plants carry water, but there are some that will carry more than others. Vines are an excellent source of water if you can get them cut open with a sharp rock. Just make sure it's not a poisonous plant first! You'll learn how to determine if something is poisonous in Chapter Three.

You've determined the type of water source you've come across and now you want to purify it. Well, there are some ways you can do this using the clothes on your body and using materials from the wilderness around you.

Boiling: Yes, boiling is the most effective way to remove viruses and bacteria from water, but it only works if you have something you can put into your fire and allow the water to boil in. If you can find a metal tin lying around the woods, boiling is not an option.

Filtering: This is the best option for those who are in an emergency situation without fire or without a container to boil their water in. How well you can filter the water you find will depend on what you can find and what you have on you in terms of clothes. The best filter foundation is a sock. It sounds disgusting but wash the sock in your water source, if you can, and try to get past the fact you're using something that was on your foot to filter your water.

Once you have the sock ready, you can use materials you're able to gather to make a filter. The first thing you want to do is make sure you find a source of carbon. This can be charcoal from your last fire, just make sure it's purely charcoal. You can also use sand, just not the sand from a river bed. Peat moss is one of the greatest water filters out there because it's a natural anti-bacterial. Regular moss will do in a pinch. And lastly, you'll want some gravel. The best way to build a filter is to put the sand in your sock first, put some moss on top of them, add some gravel, then some more moss, and sand again. Pour the water in very slowly, and the water that comes out the bottom will be purer than it was when it went in.

If you don't have a sock, you can always use a shirt, too. Just pick an item of clothing you can live without for a few hours while you purify your water. You can put it back on later.

Let's say you're desperate and you found a water source that you can confidently say is most likely free of contaminants. If you are dehydrated and you don't have the time to find the necessary materials to purify the water, then you can just drink it. Yes, there are bacteria in that water, even if it comes from a spring, but odds of it making you very sick are slim.

Finding water is one of the most important survival tips any professional could give you because the human body can only survive three days comfortably without water. After that, you're looking at serious dehydration and potentially becoming delusional. So before you find shelter, food, or anything else, find water.

Chapter Two – Quick Shelters for Any Situation

Most survivalist professionals will tell you not to leave the comforts of civilization without taking a tarp or some sort of tent with you in order to set it up when you need it, but what if you get stuck somewhere without those tools? How do you survive then? You do what your ancestors did hundreds of years ago and you use the materials around you to construct a shelter.

Take a look at some of these excellent shelters that will keep you safe, dry, and comfortable until help is able to find you.

Body-Heat Shelters: This is simply a shell shelter that creates a trapped pocket of dead air that is warmed by your body heat. When you're in an area with trees and there isn't snow, this is an excellent way to keep warm on a cool night. Body-heat shelters or debris huts are made from decomposing leaf litter and other organic debris. If you are in a snowy climate, you can make one from snow.

To make one of these simple shelters, gather a large pile of leaves, sticks, and moss from the forest floor. Then create a pocket in it large enough for you to crawl into. If it's not dirty and close enough to make your skin crawl, then the shelter is too large and you won't warm it properly with your body heat. You want to have a pine tree or similar type of tree branch in front so you can close up the hole.

A quinzee hut is an igloo that is built in a similar manner. The first step is to build te snow up to about an eight-inch depth and back it down to make a floor. Then heap some loose snow over the floor. You can pile it onto a pile of branches so it makes a mound. Allow the snow to compact for an hour or until it's hard enough you can make snowballs with it.

Then tunnel through the mound on two opposite ends in order to make a center. Fill in your unused entrance and crawl inside. Ideally, it should be narrow at your foot end with a bed long enough you can lie down. The walls and roof should be a foot thick to keep it adequately warm. Poke an air vent overhead and dig a well at the entrance to let the cold air settle in. Cut out a block of snow for the door if you can.

Open Shelters: Bough erections that will reflect your fire's heat are the best shelters to know how to construct. They are created without tools in an hour if you are in an area with some downed timber.

The pole and bough lean-to is one of the most ancient shelters created and is a single layer of materials that is a windbreak and a fire reflector. It will also protect you from a light rain or snow.

The first step is to wedge a ridgepole into the gaps of some trees growing close together. One end can rest on the ground if it needs to. Tilt the poles against the ridgepole in order to make a frame. You can strengthen it with some limber boughs through the poles at a right angle. Then thatch the lean-to with some slabs of bark or some leafy branches, weaving them into your frame. Then pat on some sod, snow, or moss to further insulate it.

The second type is an a-frame type of shelter. The pitched roof provides more shelter than a lean-to and it's able to be heated by your fire at the entrance. There is one downfall, though. You can lay down parallel to the fire in order to get even warmth. Your feet will be warm or your head will be warm.

To construct an a-frame shelter, lift up an end of your log and lash it or wedge it in a tree. Tilt the poles on either side to make an a-frame roof. Strengthen and thatch the roof just like a lean-to.

Enclosed Shelters: The next type of shelter is an enclosed shelter. They will take a few more hours than an open shelter, but they are well worth the effort. Not only it can be warmed with a small fire, but the fire will reflect off the walls and provide you with light and warmth.

The first type of enclosed shelter is a wickiup. These are one of the first types of enclosed shelters our ancestors built. They are like a tepee, but they are stronger. Wickiups are comfortable enough to serve as a long-term home if you need it to.

The first step is to tilt three poles together in a tripod and bind them near the top with a piece of your clothing, a belt, or even some bark stripped from a sapling to make rope. If you're able to find more than one pole with a 'y' at the end, tilt the others against the 'y' to eliminate the need for a rope. The second step is to tilt the other poles evenly around these three and leave a small opening at the bottom. You can thatch them together at the top for more support. Finally, add some sod as far up as you can and then leave a small gap at the top as a vent.

The second type is a wigwam. Wigwams are a more complex version of a wickiup. They are built with long, timber poles that are bent in a dome-shaped framework to maximize the interior space.

The first step to building a wigwam is to make a circle on the ground and dig holes at every two-foot interval to hold the framing poles. Then drive the butt ends of your poles into the holes and bend the smaller ends over the top, weaving them together or lashing them together to make a dome framework. The third step is to lace some thin, green poles horizontally around your framework for solidity. Finally, thatch it with branches and leave an entrance and vent hold.

The final shelter is a Salish subterranean shelter. These are not very practical unless you have something to dig with.

The first step is to dig a pit the circumference of the shelter to a depth of three feet. Build a support of tripod poles and strengthen it with some horizontally laced limbs. Then thatch it and leave a hole at the center to serve as a ladder entrance and as a vent for a smoke. Use the earth you removed to sod and insulate the walls of the shelter.

Understanding how to build a shelter without any tools will help you survive in the ultimate wilderness survival situation. It can be the difference between being alive when you're rescued or not.

Chapter Three – Finding a Food Source

Odds are, you're not going to be eating steak when you're in the middle of the wilderness trying to survive. However, there are some just as nutritious options for those who are not willing to take down large game. You just have to get past any gross factor you have about the subject. When you're actually out there and you're really hungry, it won't seem so bad.

Humans can eat just about anything that swims, crawls, flies, or walks. The first obstacle is getting past the aversion to eating any particular food source. Historically, those who have been in a starvation situation have resorted to eating anything imaginable in order to feel satisfied. Someone who ignores a healthy food source due to a personal bias will risk his or her survival.

Let's start off with protein sources as these are the best things to eat in an emergency situation. You're going to need all the protein and fat you can find.

Insects: Insects are very easily caught and they are the most abundant type of life on the plant. They provide anywhere from sixty-five to eighty percent protein compared to just twenty percent in beef. This makes insects very important when it comes to a food source. Just avoid any adults that will bite or sting. If they are hairy or brightly colored, you should avoid them, and don't try caterpillars. Anything that is commonly known to carry a disease, such as ticks, mosquitos, and flies should also be avoided.

Rotting logs are a great place to look for insects such as termites, ants, beetles, and grubs. Don't overlook an insect nest that is in or on the ground. Grassy areas like fields are a great place to search because you can easily see the insects. Boards, stones, and anything else lying on the ground are another great place to look.

Worms: Worms might really turn your stomach, but consider this, they have almost every nutrient in them you need to survive. Worms are very nutritious. Simply dig for them in some soft soil or watch for them after it rains. Place in some clean water and they will naturally rid themselves of impurities so that you can eat them raw.

Crustaceans: Freshwater shrimp can be anywhere from a quarter of a centimeter to two and a half centimeters long. They can be in a colony or they might be alone in the bottom of a pond or a lake. Crayfish are close relatives of the lobster and crab. They have a hard shell and five pairs of legs. They are active at night, but they can be located under rocks in streams.

It's best they are eaten cooked like you would a lobster. Just put them into a container in the fire and they will cook for a few minutes.

Fish: Fish are an excellent source of fat and protein, and they are not as difficult to catch as you might think. They're usually more abundant that mammals and there are ways to catch them in groups. To be successful, first you have to know their habits. Fish feed heavily before storms and are not likely to be available after a storm. When there is a heavy current, they rest in places where there's an eddy, like between rocks. They also gather where there are deep pools or overhanging brush. Pretty much anywhere they can find shelter, you will find them.

There are not any poisonous freshwater fish, but catfish do have sharp protrusions off their fins that can cause some serious damage to unprotected hands. The wounds will become infected.

Cook all freshwater fish you catch in order to avoid parasites and cook saltwater fish near reefs or in an area influenced by freshwater sources. Any marine life found out in the ocean will not have any parasites and can be consumed raw.

Certain saltwater fish will have poisonous flesh. The triggerfish, porcupine fish, cowfish, oil fish, thorn fish, jack, red snapper, and puffer are all poisonous.

Amphibians and Reptiles: Salamanders and frogs are easily found around water sources. Frogs will seldom leave the water's edge for safety purposes. They will bury into the mud and debris at the first sign of danger, so look for them there. There are some poisonous species of frogs, so avoid any brightly colored frogs or frogs with an 'x' mark on their back. Don't confuse a toad with a frog. Toads are in drier environments and will not normally be in the water. Several species of toads are poisonous and can cause death if they are eaten.

Reptiles are another excellent source of protein. They are pretty easy to catch and should be cooked. The box turtle is commonly encountered but should not be eaten. It feeds on poisonous mushrooms and can build up the toxins in its flesh. Cooking will not destroy the toxin. Avoid the hawksbill turtle in the Atlantic Ocean because it has a poisonous thorax gland. Poisonous crocodiles, alligators, snakes, and sea turtles are hazards, too.

Birds: All species of birds are safe to eat, but the flavor can vary. Fish-eating birds can be skinned in order to improve their taste. As with any animal, you have to know their habits to be able to catch them. Some can be taken from roosts at night when they are sleeping while others will need to be captured.

Nesting birds will also provide eggs. Remove all but two eggs from the clutch and mark the ones you leave. The bird will keep laying eggs to fill their clutch. Keep removing fresh eggs and leaving the ones you marked.

Mammals: We've all seen the hero in the movies who catches a deer or even a rabbit for food, but this is extremely hard to do. There are much easier food sources that do not have you expending large amounts of energy. The amount of injury a mammal can inflict can be detrimental, too. All mammals are edible, but be careful with how you catch them.

Now that you know how to find protein in order to keep yourself going, let's take a look at some plant sources. You still need to eat some plants in the wild because they will contain vitamins and nutrients you need to stay healthy. If you find you're in a long-term survivalist situation, eating plants will also help you keep your energy up while you are looking for a source of protein.

Ideally, you should know what plants are edible in the area you will be traveling to in case of an emergency, but sometimes you might not be sure. If you're unsure of a plant's edibility, then try this test.

1. Test only one part of a potential food plant at one time.
2. Separate the plan into the basic elements, roots, stems, leave, buds, and flowers.
3. Smell the food for any type of strong acid odor. Remember the smell will not indicate if it's edible or not.
4. Do not eat for eight hours before you begin the test.
5. During those eight hours when you abstain from eating, test for contact poisoning by putting a piece of the plant part you're testing on the inside of your elbow or wrist. Fifteen minutes is enough to allow for a reaction.
6. During the test period, eating nothing by mouth but water and the plant you're testing.
7. Take a small portion of a single part of the plant and prepare it the way you plan on eating it.
8. Before you put the prepared plant part into your mouth, touch a small bit to the outer surface of your lip to test for any itching or burning.
9. If there is no reaction on the lip after three minutes, put the plant part on your tongue and hold it there for fifteen minutes.

10. If there is no reaction, thoroughly chew a bit and hold it in your mouth for fifteen minutes. Don't swallow!

11. If there is no burning, numbing, itching, stinging, or any other irritation, then swallow it after fifteen minutes.

12. Wait eight hours. If any ill effects happen during this time period, induce vomiting and drink a lot of water.

13. If nothing bad happens, eat a quarter of a cup of the same plant part prepared in the same way. Wait another eight hours. If nothing bad happens, the plant part you prepared is safe to eat the way you prepared it.

It seems like a huge hassle to go through this with all the different parts of the plant and every plant you come across that you are unsure of, but it's the difference between living and dying. Consuming just a little bit of a poisonous plant without completing this test can lead to death. So it's better to be safe and a little hungry rather than sorry.

Now that you know how to find food, shelter, and water let's move on to building a fire with only what you have around you.

Chapter Four – Lighting a Fire

There are four main ways to start a fire without needing matches or any other material you cannot readily find in the wilderness. The man used to do it before we had matches, and we can surely do it again. However, it's best you practice these methods at home before you find yourself in a sticky situation.

The Hand Drill: This is the most primitive method and the most primal. It's also the hardest one to do. All you have to have is some wood, tireless hands, and some serious determination. Here's how you do it.

Build a tinder nest. It will be used to make the flame you get from the spark you'll make. Make a tinder nest out of anything you know will catch on fire easily, like some dry grass or leaves.

Next, make the notch. Cut a v-shaped notch into the fire board and make a small depression next to it.

Put the bark in the notch. The bark is going to be used to catch an ember from the friction between your spindle and fireboard.

Begin spinning. Put the spindle into the depression on the fire board. The spindle will be about two feet long for it to work right. Maintain pressure on the board and begin rolling the spindle between your two hands. Run them quickly down the spindle. Keep doing this until there are embers on the fireboard.

Then, once you see the ember, tap the fireboard to drop the ember onto the part of the bark. Relocate the bark to the nest of kindling. Then gently blow on the tinder to begin the flame.

Fire Plough: The fire plow method is very similar to the last method. You cut a groove into the fireboard, which is the track for the spindle.
Take the tip of the spindle and put it in the groove of the fireboard. Begin rubbing the tip of the spindle up and down your groove.

Have the tinder nest at the end of the fireboard so you'll plow embers into it as you rub. Once you catch one, blow the nest gently to get the fire started.

Bow Drill: This is most likely the most effective friction based method to use due to it being easier to keep the speed and pressure steady to make a fire. In addition to the spindle and the fireboard, you'll need a bow and a socket.

The socket is needed in order to put pressure on the other end of your spindle as you rotate it with the bow. It can be a stone or another piece of wood. If you use another piece of wood, try to find a harder one than you're using for the spindle. Sticks with oil and saps are excellent choices because it makes a lubricant between the spindle and socket.

The bow should be around as long as the arm. Use a flexible piece of wood with a slight curve. The string can be anything. A shoelace, some rope, or even a strip of rawhide will work. Just find something you know won't break. String up the bow and you're ready. Cut a v-shaped notch in your fireboard to make a depression attached to it in the fireboard. Put the tinder underneath the notch. Put the spindle in a loop of the bow string. Put one end of the spindle into the fireboard and apply some pressure at the other end with the socket. Use the bow to start sawing back and forth. You'll be making a rudimentary drill. The spindle should rotate fast. Keep sawing until there is an ember.
Then drop the ember into the tinder nest and blow on it to make a fire.

Flint and Steel: This is an old standby for many. It's always a good idea to keep a set with on a camping trip, but you can find rocks that will create a spark when you bang them together, too. Quartzite is a good option. Then find a piece of birch or fungus.

Grip the rock and the fungus or birch and take a hold of the rock between your thumb and forefinger. Be sure the edge is hanging out about two to three inches. Grasp the fungus or birch between your thumb and the flint.

Strike the two together to make a spark. It takes some practice, but the fungus or birch will light on fire.

While these four ways are not for the faint of heart or the beginner, they are ways you should practice in case you find yourself in a situation where you need a fire.

Lastly, in the final chapter, we'll talk about how to find help.

Chapter Five – Finding Help

When you're in the wilderness and you need to find help, there are a few different options you have with what's around you. Keep in mind that the best way to be found is to actually stay where you are. If you were in a plane crash or you simply got lost while you were hiking, you need a certain spot you get back to every day and be around that spot. It's okay to wander out a mile or two for water or food if you need them, but otherwise, stay where you are.

When you wander a mile away from where you realized you were lost, you make the search rescue party have to search three square miles in order to find you. Another mile from there and it's twelve square miles they need to search.

If you want to be found and you're planning on taking a trip, then be sure you leave a trip plan with someone who will know where you are going, what you are doing, and what time you should be back. If there is a discrepancy and they realize you are lost, they have a lot of information to give to the search party.

If you want to be found a little quicker, then there are a few things you can do in order to help the search party find you.

The first thing is to make some improvised visual signals.

Improvised Visual Signals: This is a broad category that is only really limited by your imagination and what you have at hand. The most popular one is a signal fire. However, most people make the mistake of starting a signal fire somewhere it's difficult to be seen or they use items that burn white on a cloudy day.

Throw something wet into the fire or something that will create black smoke rather than white, such as an extra jacket. Never create a fire where you know you can't put it out or allow it to get out of control. You'll make a forest fire, which will make it even harder for people to find you if you don't get caught in it first.

Improvised Audible Signals: If you don't have a whistle, then don't give up. A creative person is able to find a lot of ways they can make noise to draw attention to their location. High pitched tones can be made by using your fingers in your mouth, or you can easily carve your own whistle.

Find a hollow piece of plant material, such as a piece of bamboo or a sturdy piece of vine, and cut a hole on either end. Make sure it's not obstructed and then cut a small triangular shape on one end. Blow into it and you'll hear a high pitch noise!

Make flags with clothing, use some neon colored scraps of your clothing to wrap around some trees in the area, or begin a fire. There are plenty ways that can attract someone's attention.

Conclusion

Being caught without being prepared in the wilderness can be a frightening thing to happen. Just remember your ancestors were able to survive, and so can you. Remember that water and shelter come first, and then comes food. Tend to your needs in the order that is the most important and you will be fine until help finds you.

Thank you for reading!

www.ingramcontent.com/pod-product-compliance
Lightning Source LLC
Chambersburg PA
CBHW072013280526
45788CB00005B/2026